Sinus Infection Natural Cure

Powerful Home Remedies to Clear a Sinus Infection and Sinus Pain Permanently, Without Antibiotics

By

Kim Hilton

Sinus Infection Natural Cure

First edition. July, 2018.

Copyright © 2018 Kim Hilton

Written by Kim Hilton

Other Books by The Same Author

- Boost Your Energy Levels: 60 Natural Ways to Get Rid of Fatigue, Dizziness, Weakness, And Lack of Motivation

- How to Get Rid Of Stretch Marks Naturally

- How to Break Sugar Cravings with Nutritional Supplements: Healthy and Natural Alternatives

- The Anti-Anxiety Cookbook: Nutritional Plan to Cure Depression and Anxiety (Stress Relief and Mental Health Cookpot)

- Eating Disorder Recovery Workbook: How to Recover from Eating Disorder On Your Own (Anorexia, Bulimia Nervosa, And Binge Eating)
- 100 Health Hacks Nobody Ever Told You: Natural Tips and Tricks for Enhanced and Prudent Well-Being
- How to Lower Blood Pressure Naturally & Quickly: Powerful Tricks to Deal with Hypertension Using Supplements and Other Natural Remedies
- Reverse Type 2 Diabetes: How to Control and Prevent Diabetes Naturally

- Urinary Tract Infection Treatment: Home Remedies for Urinary Tract Infections and Prevention Methods
- Natural Treatments for Yeast Infection: How to Cure a Yeast Infection Using Home Remedies
- Itchy Skin Solution: Effective Home Remedies to Get Rid of Dry, Itchy Skin
- Top 30 Cancer-Fighting Foods: Diets and Nutritional Meal Plans to Manage, Overcome, and Prevent Cancer
- Home Remedies for Toothache: Natural Ways to Relieve Severe Toothache and Gum Pain

Table of Contents

Introduction 7

What Causes Sinusitis?.........................11

Types of Sinusitis 17

Signs and Symptoms of Sinusitis 19

How to Prevent Sinusitis 24

Natural Remedies for Sinusitis.............27

When to see a Doctor............................55

Other Books by The Same Author........56

Introduction

A sinus is an air-filled and hollow cavity in your face. There are 8 sinuses or hollow cavities in the skull and they are all connected to your nasal airways by the ostium, a narrow hole in the bone.

Humans have four pairs of cavities (making a total of eight cavities) and they are referred to as the "paranasal sinuses". "They are the frontal sinus (situated in your forehead), the sphenoid sinus (situated deep behind the ethmoids), the maxillary sinus (situated behind your cheeks), and the ethmoids sinus (situated in-between the eyes)."

The cells lining each of the sinus secrets mucus; they also secret epithelial cells and other cells like eosinophils, lymphocytes, and macrophages, these make up the solders that protect and prevent infections. They are apparently among the important elements that make up the immune system.

Sinuses have important functions in the body like humidifying and warming air you breath, insulating the surrounding structures of your eyes and the nerves also, they increase the resonance of your voice, and they also act as buffers against facial accidents and traumas, and they make your skull weigh less.

Sinus infections are also known as rhino-sinusitis or sinusitis in short, it is a common infection that is characterized by the inflammation of the cavities around the passages in your nose.

When your sinuses are healthy, they are occupied by air, but in sinusitis, the tissues lining your sinuses becomes swollen, filled with fluid and blocked. This also allows germs to grow there, thereby causing an infection.

What Causes Sinusitis?

Sinusitis is caused by viruses, these viruses damage the cells lining the sinus, and, this, in turn, will lead to inflammation. This inflammation thickens the lining and this also gives way to the obstruction of the nasal passage.

This obstruction prevents the process that expels bacteria and other harmful microbes from your sinus and nasal passage. This gives room for the bacteria and pathogens to multiply and invade the lining of your sinus, this will give rise to the symptoms of sinus infection.

Bacteria can cause sinus infection in many occasions. Bacteria that cause acute sinusitis are Staphylococcus aureus, Streptococcus pneumoniae, Moraxella catarrhalis, Haemophilus influenzae, and some anaerobic bacteria (the bacteria in question can survive without the supply of air).

In rare cases, a fungus can also cause it, especially in people with weak immune systems, like those with autoimmune diseases, HIV/AIDS, diabetes and any form of cancer. Medications that regulate the immune system also raise the risks of sinus infection.

Allergens and environmental pollutants can also give rise to a similar effect. Other causes of sinusitis are:

•	A shift in your nasal cavities, also known as deviated nasal septum

•	Common cold and other infections of the respiratory system

- Nasal polyps, these are tiny growths in the lining of your nose

- Swelling or inflammation of the lining of the nose, also known as allergic rhinitis.

- Medications that suppresses the immune system

- Drainage ducts that are blocked

- Narrowed ducts and other structural differences

- Allergies like hay fever

- Medical conditions associated with weak immune system like HIV/AIDS and acid reflux, and cystic fibrosis.

Things that can cause sinusitis in children are:

- Smoke

- Allergies

- Pacifiers

- Illnesses contacted from other kids at school or day care centers

- Drinking from a bottle while lying down on their backs

Types of Sinusitis

There are many types of sinusitis and they are usually classified based on their duration.

• Recurrent sinusitis happens man times in a year

• Acute sinusitis always starts suddenly like common cold and it lasts for two to four weeks. It has symptoms that are coldlike such as a runny nose, pressure, facial pain, and congestion.

• Chronic sinusitis lasts for more than twelve weeks despite treatments

- Subacute sinusitis 4 to 12 weeks.

Signs and Symptoms of Sinusitis

The symptoms usually depend on the type but general symptoms of acute sinusitis are:

• Nasal congestions

• Nausea

• Dizziness

• Fever

• Coughs and it worsens at night

• Your upper jaw and teeth might ache

- Sore throat

- Irritability

- Facial pressure or facial pain

- Difficulty breathing

- Halitosis (bad breath)

- Facial swellings

- Runny nose

- Inability to smell

- Pains

- Fatigue

- A stuffed-up nose

- Pressure and pain around the cheekbones and eyes

- Throat irritations

- Sensitive teeth

- Tooth pain

- Earache

- Nasal discharge that can be thick, yellow or green

Signs and symptoms of chronic sinusitis are:

- A feeling of fullness, pressure, or congestion in your face

- Headaches (sinus headaches)

- A runny nose with a discolored nasal drainage

- Bad breath

- Nasal blockage and obstructions

- Tooth ache

- Fever

- Presence of pus in your nasal cavity

- Fatigue

If left untreated, sinusitis, although in rare cases can lead to infection of the bones or skin, brain abscess, vision problem and even blindness (if it infects the socket of your eyes), complete or partial loss of smell, or meningitis.

How to Prevent Sinusitis

• Avoid breathing in dry air, use a humidifier. Make sure your clean it regularly to keep air free of mold and dirt.

• Avoid and promptly treat respiratory tract infections.

• In order to avoid infections, make washing your hands a habit after using the washroom. Use soap all the time and take the time to clean up before coming out. Do the same before meal in order to prevent the spread of diseases.

- Manage your allergies properly and avoid your triggers.

- Avoid cigarette, tobacco smoke, and other types of smoke

- Avoid harmful chemicals and other irritants.

- Another risk factor for chronic sinusitis is Asthma. So it is advised medically to be treated properly taking all the precautions.

- If you are sensitive to aspirin, avoid it because it can cause respiratory infections which raise the risk for sinusitis.

- Fortify your immune system because a suppressed immune system can make you susceptible to this infection.

Natural Remedies for Sinusitis

Water

Adequate intake of clean water and proper hydration prevents dehydration and dryness and it expels microorganisms from your body. This reduces the risks of sinusitis.

Try to drink two cups of water every two hours when you have sinusitis. You can also take lots of fruit juices, especially citrus fruit juices, smoothies, hot herbal teas, bone or chicken broth, fermented drinks and other healthy liquids.

Avoid sugary drinks because bacteria and other harmful microbes need sugar to thrive and this will worsen the symptoms of sinusitis. Avoid caffeinated drinks and alcohols because they dehydrate your body and this makes mucus thick; this thick mucus blocks your airways and also makes it inflamed.

Elderberry

This is an age long therapy for colds, sinusitis, influenza, and all kinds of infections because it has a powerful immune-boosting effect.

They fight inflammation and ease congestions, this herb also has an antiviral effect which makes it capable of treating sinusitis caused by viruses.

Cook elderberries in water till it becomes thick like syrup. Then strain it and add honey, your elderberry syrup is ready. Take few tablespoons of this every day untill you recover.

Ensure that your elderberries are properly cooked because uncooked or undercooked elderberries contain a toxic glycoside that can cause harm in your body.

Moringa

These leaves are powerful, they can clear nasal congestions and relieve other symptoms of sinusitis. To make it more potent, mix it with ginger and lemon.

Take Moringa tea daily, combined with lemon, honey and ginger to hasten healing, boost your immune system and reverse his infection.

Onions

Onions are dense in natural antibacterial, antiseptic, and antimicrobial properties. They treat a lot of infections and relieve the symptoms of sinusitis, including pressure and inflammation.

The sulfur compounds in onions are responsible for its therapeutic effects. Use an onion with a strong scent which indicates higher medicinal effects.

You can chew on it, or you juice it and take the juice in tablespoons throughout the day. You may also add chopped onions to boiling water and drink the liquid when it is hot and you can also inhale the liquid.

Boil onions in water, then blend it and sieve it properly to extract the juice, that is how to juice an onion.

Hot peppers

Chili peppers, black peppers, and cayenne peppers dissolves thick mucus, it also expels excess mucus from your system and open up your airways.

You should try and make your homemade mucus dissolving elixir by mixing apple cider vinegar with hot peppers and lemon juice. Take a teaspoon of this elixir regularly during the day to reverse this condition.

Lemon Balm

This is an effective remedy for treating the symptoms of sinusitis like a sore throat or throat irritations. It also clears congestions and opens up your airways, thereby enabling proper breathing.

Boil some leaves of lemon balm and inhale the steam, you can also gargle with this solution to treat throat infections or throat irritations. You can also drink this solution as tea.

Ginger

Ginger relieves pains and inflammation, it thins mucus and clears other symptoms of sinusitis. Take ginger tea many times daily. Mix it with lemon and raw honey.

You can inhale ginger essential oil or boil ginger and perform a face steam with the hot water. Recent studies at the

New York State University reported that sinus infection can be treated effectively using the ginger recipe, and works better than regular antibiotics.

Probiotics

These beneficial bacterial help boost your immune system, they also kill harmful microbes that can cause this infection. They eliminate them from your body and keep your system free of microbes thereby cutting the risk of sinusitis caused by bacteria and viruses.

These bacteria are presented in the gut but there are certain factors that can deplete them and when they are less in numbers, the body becomes susceptible to a lot of infections.

Research has proven that 80% of our immune system lies in the gut, and by now, you should know that your mouth, throat, nose, and sinuses are part of your digestive tract.

Increasing your levels of probiotics will help you overcome this infection and even prevent recurrence. Take lots of fermented foods and drinks, they are rich in probiotics. Examples of these are cultured yogurt, Kombucha, kefir, sauerkraut, and fermented vegetables.

Steam inhalation

This practice break up thick mucus, it expels them and opens up your respiratory airways. You can increase its effectiveness by adding essential oils like peppermint, eucalyptus, oregano, ginger or mint essential oil.

You can also add dried herbs like thyme, and other leaves of your choice. Add them to boiling water, pour the water in a bowl. Bend your head over the bowl and cover yourself with a thick towel and slowly breathe in the steam for few minutes.

Hydrogen Peroxide

This is a powerful astringent and it also kills harmful pathogens and microbes that can cause sinusitis. It prevents their growth and activities and it stops them from causing harm in your respiratory system and airways.

Use 3% hydrogen peroxide, pour this into a spray bottle. Bend over so that you can see the floor while you spray this solution into your nose. Breathe in deeply so that this solution can get to your sinuses.

Repeat this procedure every few hours.

Oregano Essential Oil

"Thymol and carvacol are the main and powerful contents of the oregano essential oil." These powerful compounds fight all types of microbes and it is a great therapy for sinusitis.

Obtain a bowl of hot water.

Add few drops of oregano oil.

Place a cotton clothing or shirt over your head and breath in the vapor coming out of the bowl.

The purpose of the cotton clothing is to prevent the vapor from escaping.

Do this for few minutes, several times daily and you will see great improvements.

Raw Honey

This is a powerful antiseptic and antimicrobial substance.

"Honey helps in getting rid of infections associated with sinus."

It also overcomes:

Inflammation caused by sinusitis

Congestion caused by sinus;

Irritation around the nasal area due to sinus;

As well as other throat infections.

Take two tablespoon of raw honey three times daily, you can mix it with lemon juice to make it more effective. Consume this mixture three times daily also.

Turmeric

This wonderful root herb treats a lot of infections because its active compound Curcumin, is a powerful antimicrobial compound. This compound also fights inflammation, pains, and relieves all the symptoms of sinusitis.

You can combine it with ginger and black pepper to boost its effectiveness. They will loosen up thick mucus that has clogged your airways, they will alleviate the pressure and make you feel great.

Pound fresh ginger and turmeric root, and if they are not available, you can make use of the powder. Add them to a cup of boiling water and leave it for few minutes. Add black pepper – a single teaspoon

Take the mixture three times; morning, afternoon and before going to bed.

Coconut Oil Pulling

You can draw out toxins, harmful microbes and germs from your oral cavity by performing oil pulling using coconut oil. This is practiced a lot in Ayurveda medicine and it also boosts the flow of lymph to your sinuses.

This act clears congestions in your airways and it prevents the buildup of mucus. It clears your nasal passages and makes you breath easily.

Rinse your mouth with coconut oil. Use 2 tablespoons and leave it for five minutes in order to penetrate through. Gaggle and rinse with pure water twice. This should be repeated daily until a significant recovery is being felt.

Grapefruit Seed Extract

Grapeseed has powerful antiviral properties, when sinusitis is caused by viruses; this remedy comes in handy because you cannot use antibiotics for viruses. This is the reason why many nasal sprays and throat sprays contain Grapefruit seed extract.

The polyphenols contained in grapefruit seed extract such as naringenin and limonoids treat sinusitis and relieve all the symptoms of this infection.

Apple Cider Vinegar

ACV helps in thinning mucus and helps eliminate excess mucus from your body. It relieves sinus pressure, headaches, inflammations, and clears congestions in your respiratory system. It works in killing bacteria aside its function in boosting the immune system.

Take two tablespoons of apple cider vinegar three times every day, you can add it to a glass of warm water if you don't like the sour taste. You can mix it with lemon juice and raw honey to boosts its effectiveness.

Vitamin C

This vitamin helps boost the immune system and help your body fight off this infection. It also kills microbes and protects your body from free radicals.

Free radicals can cause sinusitis just as smoke and air pollution. Citrus fruits, dark green leafy vegetables, and peppers are rich sources of vitamin C.

Chamomile Tea

Chamomile flower is as effective as eucalyptus in fighting infections and opening up your airways. You can drink the tea and you can also inhale it. It relieves inflammation, it boosts the immune system, expels mucus.

It relieves pain, it clears a stuffy nose and soothes irritations in your throat. Breath chamomile essential oil vapor. You can do this by simply pour a few drops in side hot water in a cup or bowl. Face the bowl and cover your head with a cotton clothing, then breath the vapor for two or three minutes.

Garlic

This is one of the best and strongest antibiotics provided by Mother Nature. It treats a lot of infections like sinusitis; regular ingestion of garlic prevents this infection in the first place.

It also boosts your immune system and kills harmful microbes. It hastens recovery and prevents recurrence. Take fresh cloves of garlic daily.

Fortunately, the garlic powder and other supplements alike can be easily found at the grocery store. Health stores also make supplements available for convenience sake.

Peppermint Tea

An active phytochemical present is peppermint is menthol, it thins mucus and expels excess mucus from the body. It is a natural and effective expectorant and decongestant.

Add some drops of peppermint essential oil into a bowl of boiling water and inhale the steam.

Peppermint tea also plays a significant role when it comes clearing sinusitis from the throat.

Get a cup of a boiled hot water.

Add peppermint leaves to the cup (a few drops will do).

Allow it to stay for 10 minutes.

Strain it, add raw honey and then try drinking it when hot so that you will get fast relief from sinusitis.

Echinacea

This is an immune boosting herb that can also fight and eliminate a wide range of microbes. Traditional healers use it in treating sinusitis, respiratory infections, and other types of infections.

It contains many phytochemicals that fight viruses and bacteria, and it also relieves inflammation and pains. You can take the tea or the capsules.

Pineapples

Pineapples and unsweetened pineapple juice can help you fight sinusitis because this sweet fruit contains an enzyme called bromelain. This enzyme fights inflammation and relieves all the symptoms of sinusitis.

Eat lots of fresh pineapples and take homemade unsweetened pineapple juice daily.

Bromelain supplements are available, but it can lead to toxicity when taken in excess and it also interacts with some medications like blood thinners and anti-hypertensive drugs.

Neti Pot

Rinsing your nostrils with saline solution using a neti pot is an effective treatment for sinusitis and respiratory infections. The process of using neti pot is called "nasal irrigation", it even eliminates the symptoms of chronic sinusitis.

It reduces headaches, recurrence, and it improves the way you feel when having sinusitis. You can make your own saline solution at home by adding a tablespoon of table salt to a cup of warm water. Your

saline solution is ready.

When to see a Doctor

Please, see a doctor immediately if you observe any of the following symptoms:

- A stiff neck

- A high body temperature

- Changes in vision like blurred vision or double vision

- Severe headache

- Redness or swellings around your eyes

- Confusion

Other Books by The Same Author

- Boost Your Energy Levels: 60 Natural Ways to Get Rid of Fatigue, Dizziness, Weakness, And Lack of Motivation

- How to Get Rid Of Stretch Marks Naturally

- How to Break Sugar Cravings with Nutritional Supplements: Healthy and Natural Alternatives

- The Anti-Anxiety Cookbook: Nutritional Plan to Cure Depression and Anxiety (Stress Relief and Mental Health Cookpot)

- [Eating Disorder Recovery Workbook: How to Recover from Eating Disorder On Your Own (Anorexia, Bulimia Nervosa, And Binge Eating)](#)
- [100 Health Hacks Nobody Ever Told You: Natural Tips and Tricks for Enhanced and Prudent Well-Being](#)
- [How to Lower Blood Pressure Naturally & Quickly: Powerful Tricks to Deal with Hypertension Using Supplements and Other Natural Remedies](#)
- [Reverse Type 2 Diabetes: How to Control and Prevent Diabetes Naturally](#)

- Urinary Tract Infection Treatment: Home Remedies for Urinary Tract Infections and Prevention Methods
- Natural Treatments for Yeast Infection: How to Cure a Yeast Infection Using Home Remedies
- Itchy Skin Solution: Effective Home Remedies to Get Rid of Dry, Itchy Skin
- Top 30 Cancer-Fighting Foods: Diets and Nutritional Meal Plans to Manage, Overcome, and Prevent Cancer
- Home Remedies for Toothache: Natural Ways to Relieve Severe Toothache and Gum Pain